Along the Road—Tales of the Journey

Along the Road—Tales of the Journey

A Life Review Workbook for Individuals and Groups

N. Thomas Johnson-Medland, CSJ, OSL

RESOURCE *Publications* · Eugene, Oregon

ALONG THE ROAD—TALES OF THE JOURNEY
A Life Review Workbook for Individuals and Groups

Copyright © 2011 N. Thomas Johnson-Medland. All rights reserved. Except for brief quotations in critical publications or reviews, no part of this book may be reproduced in any manner without prior written permission from the publisher. Write: Permissions, Wipf and Stock Publishers, 199 W. 8th Ave., Suite 3, Eugene, OR 97401.

Wipf & Stock
An Imprint of Wipf and Stock Publishers
199 W. 8th Ave., Suite 3
Eugene, OR 97401
www.wipfandstock.com

ISBN 13: 978-1-61097-196-6

Manufactured in the U.S.A.

All scripture quotations, unless otherwise indicated, are taken from the Holy Bible, New International Version®, NIV®. Copyright ©1973, 1978, 1984 by Biblica, Inc.™ Used by permission of Zondervan. All rights reserved worldwide.

This book is dedicated to all the patients and families that have worked through the tough issues facing them while on hospice care; to the Leadership Team of Lighthouse Hospice in Cherry Hill, New Jersey whose love, dedication, and hard work became a refining and deepening process in my life; and to Elisabeth Kubler-Ross—the one who lit the lamp for all of us in hospice and end-of-life work.

*Live, so you do not have to look back and say:
"God, how I have wasted my life."*

—Elisabeth Kübler-Ross

Contents

Acknowledgments ix
How to use this book xi
When I have finished this book xiii
Introduction xv

1 Family 1

2 Friends 63

3 Faith 85

4 My Life 111

5 Pearls of Wisdom 153

6 Notes and Pictures 161

7 Feelings surrounding illness and death 177

8 Funeral Plans 207

9 Elisabeth Kübler-Ross 215

Afterward 219

Acknowledgments

A SPECIAL THANKS TO the Lighthouse Foundation of New Jersey and its board members Sandra L. Cunningham, Susan Curry, and Michelle Boyd, RN., for the writing and research grant they made available for the completion of this workbook. Without their investment in this project I would never have been able to see it through to completion.

I would also like to thank all of my friends in hospice over the years from: Heritage Hospice, Caring Hospice, Lighthouse Hospice, NHPCO, and NJHPCO. The work we were able to do and are still able to do is always a blessing and so fulfilling. It has been my pleasure working with you all; giving from our hearts to each other, to the dying, and to their loved ones. As we know, it is still nothing compared to the precious gift our patients and their families give us—the gift of teaching us how to live. May our work honor their memories.

Ira Byock, MD and Karen Taylor-Good, thanks for your ongoing contributions to the larger end-of-life community. Like Elisabeth (Kübler-Ross), you inspire us to work diligently with integrity, feeling, and a deep seated compassion - tending the lives of all those we touch. Without your flames, the hospice community would be less warm and inviting.

Thank you also to the countless organizations that seek to remediate suffering at end-of-life. To all of the Cancer Coalitions of New Jersey (and across the country), the hospices, hospitals, and care facilities, WHYY Wider Horizons and other grass roots advocacy organizations—may your work continue to be a bridge by which others may cross over to compassion and a cessation of suffering.

Finally, thank you to my dear sister in end-of-life care, Elisabeth Kübler-Ross. The phone calls we shared over the years and the few days toward the end have bolstered and informed the end-of-life writing that I have done and the visits I have made. Without your persistent reminder to find a home for this workbook and to keep at the task of producing materials to help support the work of caring for the dying, I would have languished on the vine a long time ago. I am so glad you were able to find your rest. Thank you for the milestones and markers you left for us.

How to use this book

THIS BOOK IS INTENDED for individual and or group use. It is something that you can go through and fill out for yourself and by yourself. You can also fill this out with your family and loved ones as a way of telling the stories while you are recording them. You can use it to lead a discussion group or support group in either a religious or a secular environment.

It is also something that end-of-life professionals and caregivers will want to use to shape the nature of your meetings with patients and families. You can plan to go over a few items or sections at a time in order to develop the work you are doing together—using the workbook as a springboard. The topics dovetail nicely into care-plans identifying life review, decreased isolation, funeral planning, and spiritual closure or existential searching.

When a patient or a loved-one is non-responsive, this workbook may be a valuable guidebook for sharing time in their presence. You can engage in family meetings and life review while in the presence of your unresponsive patient or loved-one. One of the things we have learned from hospice care is that nonresponsive does not mean unaware. People always want to know that those around them are processing what is going on.

The workbook's greatest power will be found in filling it out long before anyone enters the end-of-life phase represented by what culture and insurance companies have termed "hospice care". However, this book is designed to use anywhere along the life continuum. If more people digested the material represented here (garnered from over 15 years of working on end-of-life issues with patients, families and professionals) we could be assured of a more comprehensive cultural understanding of death and dying as well as a more conscious personal approach to living, grieving, and dying.

However it is used, it is critical that it be shared or made available to friends and family once it is completed. You will need to appoint someone to care for the stories and also to see that it is made available to those who may benefit from what it holds.

*When I have finished this book, or
upon my death, I would like
this book to go to:*

_____

*Please be sure to share my tales
with the people I love and
have been loved by.*

THANK YOU!

SIGNED: _____
   DATE: _____

Introduction

THE FIRST FIVE YEARS of our marriage, my wife and I were fortunate to work crazy jobs. We worked in social services caring for abused and neglected children at a residential treatment facility. Care had to be provided around the clock. This meant working all sorts of hours. It also meant creative scheduling.

We were both supervisors, so we often had to work shifts we could not cover otherwise. Many times we worked the weekends and the holidays. We had to work midnight until morning. We had to work morning until night.

We were at the bottom of the pile in terms of socially understood professions, but we loved providing care for distressed and abused individuals. Providing compassion to folks who had not received a lot of it was filled with difficulty and joy. It helped heal the wounds in the hearts of those we cared for. It helped heal wounds in our own hearts as well. Something opens up inside of you—that begins to nourish you—when you apply yourself to difficult circumstances.

It gave us a basis for understanding the grand grace and mercy that was afoot in life if we listened for it—the grace and mercy that comes from plugging into your woundedness. The hard work made us understand the value of having time off. We learned how to make the best use of our downtime; to play hard, too.

One of the fortunate parts of our jobs was having Mondays off. This does not seem too brilliant a fortune. Having Monday's off meant everyone else was working. There was no one else around. There was never any waiting in lines or waiting to get a table at a restaurant. There was also no one else to do anything with, because they were all at work. We had to learn to spend time together alone.

We got into the habit of going hiking together—by ourselves. We had undivided time together; something which we have not had the luxury of sharing until recently—22 years later. Every Monday we would

xv

map out a portion of a trail and either hike it in a loop—three miles out and then three back. Or, we would hike out 6-8 miles and hitchhike back to our car. Either way, we were guaranteed a full day of hiking together.

Some days this was a good thing, other days a real trial. Some days we laughed and laughed and discovered deep pieces of each other's souls. Some days we just fought or got quiet. One thing we learned about life was that staying in it for the long haul with each other was going to be tough. It would take work.

Sometimes you got something out of the hike. Sometimes you just got the hike. Some days you could expect rich conversation. Some days you could not expect conversation or anything else - just the view. You were side by side on the journey—nothing else.

There would be times when the trail would get tough, or the discussion would get tough and there would be no way to stop and go home. We often had to persevere through difficult times because there was no option for us at that moment. We were stuck on the trail—with each other. Sometimes painful words turned to silence and then back to words. Sometimes rain turned to snow and then back to rain. Sometimes the joy of each other's company was an awesome experience of union and mercy.

We learned the value of stories. We talked and talked and talked on these hikes. We wove in and out of family lore and tales, up and over ideas and philosophies, in and out of what we felt we could and could not promise each other. Every turn and bend provided a new vista for our eyes, opening our hearts to whole new layers and dimensions—as what lay before us prompted us to wander through the landscape of what lay inside us as well.

One of the most memorable walks we had involved the creation of the first line of a poem. We both love to write. It happened that on this crisp fall morning we walked past a field that had just had a trench dug through it. The sights, sounds, and smells were autumnal beyond compare. It was the quintessential fall day.

We hiked along the field. Apparently, some sort of utility was going to be laid in the field for an up and coming housing development. Greens, and reds, and yellows, and gold surrounded the field. Autumn was working her magic and the leaves were bursting with color.

Adding to the beauty of the crisp air and the pallet of color was the smell of sassafras and earth. It seems the ditch had been scored through a grove of sassafras trees. The aroma of the torn open roots and dirt filled the air.

We played with words for the opening of a poem or story that was steeped in the richness of the moment. We ended up with, "Bury me in a sassafras grave." We both have threatened through the years to copyright and use this phrase in our magnum opus. Some twenty two years later, I am the first to put it in print—at least published print. But, its rendering still opens my heart to the power of that fall day and the exquisite glory of smelling loam and root with my lovely wife.

It was and is a beautiful line. It was and is a beautiful image. The whole point lies in the notion that when we hike, or walk or amble together we are able to unearth who we are and create ways of being together. Playfully, we are able to experience the richness of life and its meaning as we amble and wander. Hiking is a metaphor for life. It is an icon for uncovering meaning in our days. And, in the moments of journeying together, we create a common language that holds a robust meaning able to decorate and reveal our lives. Just like a sassafras grave.

Wandering along the road of this life's journey can produce fashionable words and images that are formed over the many days into tales and maps. This notion is not just applicable to situations in which we actually hike, walk or amble. It is clearly a metaphor for living in proximity with other people. Our lives are a hike, a walk, and an amble with others and among the immensity of all creation.

We are heading out, along the road, with those gathered about us. We have before us, and behind us, a stretch of road and trail that we have walked together or are planning on walking. There have been stories told, philosophies and beliefs drawn up and mapped out, commitments and promises made.

That is what this book is about. It is about everything in the journey you are taking. It is about the stories, philosophies, beliefs, commitments and promises. It is about the tales told while hiking the road of your life. Dreams and hopes are spun, disappointments and agony are lived. It is all part of the trail. It is all part of the road and the tales of the journey.

This workbook is here to help you smelt out the tales of your ambling. It is here to help you put down the places you have been, the miles you have covered. These notes are important for those who are all about you. Your life informs everyone else who has touched you. As the "Phantom DNA" experiments of Dr Poponin revealed; once a life comes into contact with another, it will always have a connection, even when it is apparently physically absent. What is the truth behind local and non-local forms of reality and life?

These tales and reflections that you record here will be the sparks that ignite and illumine the way for your traveling partners and fellow journeyers. These stories and yarns will be the sparks that give imagination a chance to blaze into illuminating fire. These reflections will be a light to the path of others. So, go at them with a poetic relish for words and the telling.

The one great mystery I love to get trapped in is the mystery of our lives and our stories. It is a real circle of joy and chaos that nourishes and warms us. Does the biological hardwiring of our lives affect the stories we live and create or, do the stories we live and create alter and arrange the hardwiring of our biology? I wonder.

I would have to agree with my wife's favorite maxim. It is not a case of "either or" but a case of "both and." They are both wrapped around each other. Not one or the other, but both. Our lives and the stories we live out, affect our bodies and the bodies of those we journey with. Our bodies affect the lives we live and the stories we live out as well.

Along the Road—Tales of the Journey is a practical guide for patients and families going through some very serious and difficult issues. It is here to enable focus and meaning in a time that is fraught with confusion and pain. It is also for people who are not involved in hospice; people that recognize the value of keeping track of the journey for others to have "in case" they should suddenly be removed from the trail of life. It is for those who recognize the personal value in journaling their days for self reflection and perspective. It is for those who know they are dying, and for those whose dying is "a long ways off".

This workbook is a series of prompts that will help you notice the trail markers in your life and journey. It is a guidebook that you will write to show others the path you have taken. It is a place to reveal who you are so others may learn. So, go at it with a poetic relish for words and the telling.

I am so blessed to have journeyed with over 1500 patients and families in my years of hospice work. Each person has vilified the belief that we are all on a trail that is clearly related to who we are. Where we have been is wrapped around who we are and both are great things to share around a campfire—the "Great Campfire of Life".

There are a number of ways you can do the work in this workbook. It is strongly suggested to do it with someone else. This book should not be something you do in privacy and then squirrel away somewhere. No, this is meant to help families and friends emerge from joy and pain, connected to their strengths and gifts. It is a communal act, a ritual of love and unity. It is a yarn to be shared around the fires of life. It is also meant to be a starting place for the telling of the tales of your life journey.

My hope is that you will work on these pages with friends, spouses, partners, children, grandchildren, hospice and medical professionals, volunteers and all those who are a part of your circle of living. My hope is that you will involve some people that may help you heal as you do the work: a therapist, a social worker, a spiritual friend or clergy.

Our living and our dying do not really belong to us alone. We are members of a larger journey. Our living and our dying are something that is a part of the community—part of what the community must work through. For, no man is an island—neither is a woman.

This workbook is about bringing some of the truths of life and death to the surface so we can look at them, feel them, and celebrate them with laughter and tears. It is about following the path we have forded and sharing its events with those in our midst. It is a homecoming.

Of course this workbook is to be left behind for those who follow you on this road of life. There are so many things that people want to remember about you.

If you are working on this book at the end-of-life, the frequency with which you speak to people now, and the ease with which you speak to them now will change as time moves on. You will weaken and lose your abilities over time. This is a chance to put down the things you want people to remember and know, while you still have access to them and access to sharing them.

You may want to choose one person to have this book when you are finished, or you may want to hold on to it until you leave this physical existence. Either way, make sure you designate a person that should be the keeper of the stories. There is a space for this in these pages.

This does not mean no one else should see it. This means the keeper of the stories will always know where the tales are. This person should not be the only one involved in assisting you to mark out the stories. This is your book and your story, involve as many people as you care to—employ great freedom and love in making your map.

Pace yourself on the work to be done. Don't try to rush and do it all in a day or a weekend. Your mind and your heart can only process so much information at one time.

One day you may be really foggy on what happened in childhood, but two days later, memories and feelings may flow freely. Go gently through this beautiful work. Go back again and again.

One of my hopes is that you will find a deep and abiding sense of awe and radical amazement when you look over your life. We very rarely get the chance to see the bird's eye view of our own life. Relish that view; it is grand.

This will not abolish the sadness that often accompanies life review (at end-of-life) as you seek closure to a life lived, but it will greatly augment and offset the pain. Our lives, like most other things, are larger and more complex than we can either imagine or remember. Bask in the depth of your days here and in your journey along the road.

I am not naïve. There are painful and horrible things that have happened to you, as well as good. Some of them may have been already healed. Some of them may still need some healing. Remember, our lives are not only recordings of events, but very strong and powerful emotions as well.

If there are people that you need to forgive, do not shy away from the task at hand. If you need to be forgiven, ask. Mend what you can; while you can.

When mending is impossible, or others do not respond, close your eyes and offer your intention to mend to that person, asking them in your heart to accept this intention as reparation. Then, let go of what pieces you held in the turmoil. If it was anger, or hurt, or guilt, or sadness let it go with the intention of love. As we know, sometimes intention toward good is the best we can offer or have.

I would also recommend collecting photos and other memorabilia that go along with the memories you are recording. Find a grand album or a fancy treasure-box to keep them in. Be sure to label them so people can make the connections. When you are discussing your family and friendships, make sure you have pictures or letters of these folks stored away. When you are telling about that favorite trip, be sure a few postcards are stored as well.

May the work you do be a garden of beauty and a path of joy for you and for those you love. Wander amid the trail of your journey. And remember, "All that wander are not lost." Share the wanderings of your life and deepen the lives of those you love.

1

Family

IF THERE IS ANYTHING that has been consistent throughout our lives and our travels it has been the presence of family. And, although family may often present conflicts and difficulties that cause us to grow under pressure, there are moments of joy and relief that come from the immediate presence of those with whom we share our family ties. All of it is glommed together into the second and deepest matrix of community (the first being the matrix of the mother-bond) that we experience as human beings.

Your stories may be about "family of choice" rather than "family of birth" if you have bonded more deeply with people that fulfill familial roles rather than actual "blood". Sometimes we develop these relationships out of necessity, because there are no other options, sometimes as a means of survival. In either case use the space as best represents your life connections.

The way we have woven family into our lives allows others to gain a glimpse of who we are and where we have been. Some days we may be inextricably bound to our families; while other days we may seek the solitude of distance to mend or grow.

This section is meant to help you set down the memories you have of your family. There will be places for you to fill out things you want them to know that perhaps you do not feel strong enough to communicate, or do not feel you have enough time to do in person. These pages are in no way meant to provide you with a chance to neglect saying something you should say face-to-face. But they are meant to be a place to set down what you think and feel while you are working on how to say what it is you feel needs to be said.

Use these stories as a starting place for conversations when you are together with those you love. You know how there are often uncomfortable gaps in the conversations of life (especially since you have become sick if you are terminally ill). Your stories will give courage and focus to your times together; filling in those gaps with connective tales.

FAMILY TREE

On these next few pages jot down what you can remember of the family tree. Reach back as far as you can in your mind to come up with names of family members. Try to include dates of births and deaths when you can. Remember to use "=" between people that are married and then to list their children under them. You may want to use a pencil on this section—just in case you need to make additions or corrections.

MEMORIES OF BIRTHS

Write out what you can about the various births in your family. Were there guests present? Did a priest or rabbi come? Do you remember the weather? Do any special gifts come to mind? How about first impressions of the baby? Be sure to identify how the person you remember fits into the family scheme of things: "my second cousin on my Mother's side."

MEMORIES OF DEATHS

Use this space to record your memories of family deaths. Were there people present? What led up to the death? Were there any special events surrounding the death or special statements? Where is the person buried? What do you remember about them? What was their legacy? What did they teach you or impart to you?

Family 11

ALONG THE ROAD—TALES OF THE JOURNEY

SOME OF THE LARGER FAMILY MEMORIES

What big memories do you have from your family? Try to capture the memory by listing specifics that make it so memorable?

Special trips

Family

Favorite foods

Funny stories

Favorite people

Family 23

ALONG THE ROAD—TALES OF THE JOURNEY

Favorite gatherings and gathering places

Family

Secret recipes

Family 29

THINGS YOUR FAMILY TAUGHT YOU

What values and special lessons do you remember learning from your family? This includes things your grand-pop may have taught you on his knee, or it may be things that you learned from dealing with your family. How about that time you learned about giving to someone in need when you were struggling to get by yourselves?

Family 31

LETTERS TO YOUR FAMILY

This space is for letters to people you want to contact. Let them know how you feel and do not be afraid to talk about your love for them. This is not just for the living, but also for people who have died. There may be something you want to write to them, like your appreciation to them for taking you to the beach every summer, and teaching you how to crab. Make sure that if they are living you copy these letters and mail them. Deepen your bonds while alive.

ETHICAL WILLS

This space is for you to write out things you want to leave for people. These things are not material possessions. They are things that live inside of us; powerful and monumental images or feelings. Ethical wills include things like special memories you have of a person, gifts you admire in people which they should know about. Maybe you want your nephew to have your sense of humor or for your son to never forget the view of the mountains from your cabin. You give whatever image or memory you want your loved ones to have. These things will live on with greater meaning than most heirlooms we can touch. They will shape character and instill dignity. Just list the names and what you "will" for them.

OTHER FAMILY MEMORABILIA

Describe your parents

Describe your spouse/life partner

Family 43

Describe your wedding or significant meeting event

Describe your children or your intimate family group

*Describe other family members
(aunts/uncles, cousins, grandparents/children)*

What blessings have come from being in family

What difficulties have come from being in family

Other things there was no space for

2

Friends

As with family, friends share a significant role in our lives. I like to think of friends as our "family of choice". When we are born into our families, we have no choice about the players. But, our friends we choose. And, we choose how close we will let each friend into our lives and hearts. Some friends come in very close to us, while others remain on the periphery. Celebrate these friendships in these pages. You may have begun discussions about these friends in the family section if your "family of birth" is not really a major part of your journey, add to those stories here.

This section is meant to help you set down the memories you have of your friends. There will be places for you to fill out things you want them to know that perhaps you do not feel strong enough to communicate, or do not feel you have enough time to do in person. These pages are in no way meant to provide you with a chance to neglect saying something you should say face-to-face. But they are meant to be a place to set down what you think and feel while you are working on how to say what it is you feel needs to be said.

Use these stories as a starting place for conversations when you are together with those you love. You know how there are often uncomfortable gaps in the conversations of life (especially since you have become sick if you are terminally ill). Your stories will give courage and focus to your times together; filling in those gaps with connective tales.

LIST YOUR CLOSEST FRIENDS AND HOW YOU MET

WHAT THINGS HAVE YOU DONE WITH THESE FRIENDS

ALONG THE ROAD—TALES OF THE JOURNEY
WHAT HAVE YOU LEARNED FROM YOUR FRIENDS

WHAT KEY STORIES AND MEMORIES OF FRIENDSHIP DO YOU WANT TO SHARE

LETTERS TO YOUR FRIENDS

This space is for letters to people you want to contact. Let them know how you feel and do not be afraid to talk about your love for them. This is not just for the living, but also for people who have died. There may be something you want to write to them, like your appreciation to them for taking you to the beach every summer, and teaching you how to crab. Make sure that if they are living you copy these letters and mail them. Deepen your bonds while alive.

ETHICAL WILLS

This space is for you to write out things you want to leave for people. These things are not material possessions. They are things that live inside of us; powerful and monumental images or feelings. Ethical wills include things like special memories you have of a person, gifts you admire in people which they should know about. Maybe you want your nephew to have your sense of humor or for your son to never forget the view of the mountains from your cabin. You give whatever image or memory you want your loved ones to have. These things will live on with greater meaning than most heirlooms we can touch. They will shape character and instill dignity. Just list the names and what you "will" for them.

PRINCIPLES THAT FRIENDSHIP HAS TAUGHT YOU

3

Faith

Faith or belief in God—or a Higher Power—is vital for many people. Often, as we go through our lives, some of our values and beliefs change. This space is for you to describe your faith and beliefs and where you have been with them. Be sure to note if things changed from when you were a child until this point in your life. If you know why, make sure to include that, too.

WHAT ARE YOUR BELIEFS ABOUT GOD
OR A HIGHER POWER

Faith

HOW WOULD YOU DESCRIBE GOD

WHAT FAVORITE RELIGIOUS WRITINGS DO YOU READ OFTEN

ALONG THE ROAD—TALES OF THE JOURNEY
FAVORITE HYMNS AND PRAYERS

WHO ARE YOUR REVERED TEACHERS OR SAINTS

FOND MEMORIES OF MAJOR EVENTS CELEBRATED IN A RELIGIOUS COMMUNITY

HOW HAS ILLNESS CHANGED YOUR FAITH OR BELIEFS IN GOD

WHAT ARE YOUR HOPES FOR LIFE AFTER DEATH

HOW HAS YOUR FAITH BEEN A SUPPORT OR COMFORT THROUGHOUT YOUR LIFE

ALONG THE ROAD—TALES OF THE JOURNEY
PLACES YOU HAVE WORSHIPPED

WHAT HAS YOUR FAITH TAUGHT YOU ABOUT LIVING

WHAT HAVE YOU LEARNED ABOUT LOVE

WHAT HAVE YOU LEARNED ABOUT FORGIVENESS

WHAT HAVE YOU LEARNED ABOUT PRAYER

WHAT DO YOU BELIEVE ABOUT DEATH

WHO HAVE BEEN YOUR CLOSE SPIRITUAL FRIENDS AND MENTORS

WHAT HAVE THESE FRIENDS AND MENTORS TAUGHT YOU

WHAT SPECIAL "THEOPHANIES" ("AH-HA" MOMENTS OR REVELATIONS) HAVE YOU HAD

4

My Life

Try to flesh out where you have been throughout your life. These images and stories will be important in the handing down of values and meaning of not only your life, but also of the greater picture that your life fits into and is a part of.

We sometimes forget the value that people find in hearing where we have been and what we have done. So, take pride in answering the pieces of this section, knowing that people will find growth in the places you have been. Each of our journeys has so much to offer.

TALK ABOUT YOUR CHILDHOOD

WHERE HAVE YOU LIVED

My Life

WHAT SCHOOLS AND GROUPS HAVE YOU BEEN A PART OF

WHAT HAVE BEEN YOUR HOPES AND DREAMS THROUGHOUT LIFE

WHAT ACCOMPLISHMENTS DO YOU REMEMBER MOST

HAS YOUR LIFE HAD MAJOR THEMES

WHAT HAVE YOU BEEN UNABLE TO ACCOMPLISH

LIST HIGH POINTS

LIST LOW POINTS

WHAT ARE YOUR FAVORITES

Colors

Cars

Food

Ice cream

Songs

Movies

Actors

Books

Authors

People

Holidays

Trips

Ways to dress

Gifts you received

Gifts you gave

ALONG THE ROAD—TALES OF THE JOURNEY

Memories

Nighttime Dreams

List other favorites

LIST THE MOST IMPORTANT MEMORIES ABOUT YOU
THAT YOU DON'T WANT TO BE FORGOTTEN

WHAT ARE YOUR GREATEST STRENGTHS AND GIFTS

LIST JOBS YOU HAVE HAD

MEMORABLE WORK EXPERIENCES

IMPORTANT WORK VALUES YOU HAVE LEARNED

MEMORABLE CO-WORKERS AND IMPORTANT THINGS THEY TAUGHT YOU

THINGS THAT MAKE YOU LAUGH

FUNNY THINGS YOU REMEMBER DOING

THINGS THAT MAKE YOU CRY

OTHER THINGS YOU DID NOT HAVE SPACE FOR

5

Pearls of Wisdom

Use these pages to leave any "Pearls of Wisdom" you have found throughout life. These should be things (wisdom-statements or aphorisms) that have made your life different or changed your life drastically. These can be silly things like, "Floss daily. You only get one set of teeth." Or, serious like, "Hold your kids as often as you can." Be a sage about this portion. Return to it often as you remember sage advice or stumble upon "nuggets of truth" in your daily ambling and reading. What you leave will be strung together and used to adorn the inner life and outer character of those you love.

-

-

-

-

-

-

-

-

-

-

-

-

-

-

-

-

-

-

-

-

-

-

-

-

-

-

-

-

-

-

-

-

-

-

-

-

-

-

-

-

-

-

-

160 ALONG THE ROAD—TALES OF THE JOURNEY

•

•

•

•

•

•

6

Notes and Pictures

These pages are for special cards, notes, and pictures from those around you. They are for you to hold on to and look at often. They are for others to cherish. They may be from this portion of your life or any other part of your life. I would recommend having an album or a treasure-box to collect the majority of these things in, but keep the most special ones here, close to your hard work. Glue or tape them in place so they do not get lost.

Notes and Pictures

Notes and Pictures

Notes and Pictures 175

7

Feelings surrounding illness and death

This portion of the workbook may be difficult to fill out. The reason it has been included is that there are many feelings that emerge as you review your life and consider that it will one day be over (at least as we now know it).

These issues will be larger and more all pervasive if death is imminent or you are on hospice care. This may be the only place you have to process these feelings.

We hope these pages will set you free into looking at some of the feelings that get bottled up in us surrounding illness and death. As you write these things out, and share them with the people helping you, you will notice a sense of relief. Some of this relief comes from just getting the feelings out. Some of this relief comes from creating opportunities to discuss these feelings further—utilizing the support of clergy, volunteers, social work staff, family and friends. Our lives are always seeking further unfolding and resolution.

In addition to offering you a place to vent feelings, this section will be valuable for others in your life. Death is a quiet subject in our lives as individuals and a society. Very rarely do we know how to "feel around dying". We fear sharing experiences from our own perceptions of death and our own dying.

Your sharing of these feelings may be one of the greatest gifts you have to give to those who care for and about you. It may be the greatest gift you give to yourself. Sometimes we have questions about the tragic death of a loved one that we never got to make sense out of - we carry these issues all through our lives looking for a time and place to look at them. Sometimes it is a simple statement of relief that we never got to bear witness to. Other times it is the chance to question why things happen.

Go gently into your heart.

WHAT DEATHS DO YOU REMEMBER MOST

ARE THERE ANY QUESTIONS OR COMMENTS YOU HAVE
ABOUT THOSE DEATHS

TALK ABOUT YOUR EXPERIENCES WITH ILLNESS AND DISEASE

TALK ABOUT YOUR CURRENT LIVING WITH A TERMINAL ILLNESS

When did you get sick

How did you find out about your illness

What kinds of physical and emotional changes have you been through

How did things go for you when you found out your illness was terminal

How about since then

WHAT HAS GOTTEN YOU THROUGH THE DIFFICULT FEELINGS

WHAT HAVE YOUR FEELINGS SHOWN YOU

HAVE YOU LEARNED ANYTHING FROM BEING ILL

WHAT FEELINGS ARE HARDEST TO FACE

WHAT FEELINGS HAVE BEEN ENDEARING

HOW DO YOU FEEL ABOUT DEATH

WHAT ARE YOUR FEARS

WHAT DO YOU LOOK FORWARD TO ON A DAILY BASIS

WHAT HAVE BEEN YOUR JOYS SINCE YOUR ILLNESS

Feelings surrounding illness and death 193

TALK ABOUT DREAMS YOU HAVE HAD DURING SLEEP

ALONG THE ROAD—TALES OF THE JOURNEY
HAVE YOU HAD ANY UNUSUAL OCCURRENCES

WHAT DO YOU WANT TO TELL OTHER PEOPLE ABOUT LIVING AND DYING

HOW DO YOU FEEL ABOUT YOUR CARE

HOW DO YOU FEEL ABOUT THOSE WHO COME TO SEE YOU

HOW DO YOU FEEL ABOUT THE LIFE YOU HAVE LIVED

HAVE ANY OF YOUR FEELINGS
ABOUT DEATH CHANGED AND HOW

HOW HAVE YOU LEARNED TO ALLEVIATE SUFFERING AND PAIN (PHYSICALLY/EMOTIONALLY)

ANYTHING ELSE THERE HAS BEEN NO ROOM FOR

8

Funeral Plans

There may be some specific things you want to happen after you die. Take the time to let people know what they are. Include your family or spiritual care provider in this portion so you get some help and perspective from others.

ARE THERE RELIGIOUS RITES YOU WOULD LIKE JUST PRIOR TO DEATH OR JUST AFTER DEATH

HOW DO YOU WANT YOUR BODY TO BE INTERRED (BURIAL OR CREMATION)

Any specific instructions on cremation or the interment

What would you like to be wearing

WHAT HYMNS OR MUSIC
WOULD YOU LIKE THERE TO BE AT YOUR SERVICE

HOW ABOUT READINGS FROM SCRIPTURES OR OTHER TEXTS

WHAT WOULD YOU LIKE THE SERVICE TO BE LIKE

What funeral home do you wish to use

What clergy

Do you want anyone else to speak

Are there any specific or special prayers you want used

Do you have any other special comments, directions, or requests

Any special photos you want on hand that day

Anything you want to say to those who will gather

DID YOU PLAN TO DONATE ANY ORGANS

If so, list specific details: phone numbers or agencies, etc.

DO YOU OWN A BURIAL PLOT AND IF SO, WHERE

ANYTHING ELSE

9

Elisabeth Kübler-Ross

THE FIRST CONVERSATION I had with Elisabeth should have clued me in to who she was and how she would find a place in my heart. She was rough and tumble—an iconoclast. I loved that and still do.

I was asking her what message she would have me share with pastoral care providers at an upcoming hospice clergy luncheon. She swiftly responded, "Scare the HELL out of them! Tell them to forget their books and formula prayers and just go in to the rooms of the dying and LISTEN!" "JUST LISTEN!"

That is exactly what I shared with them. I told them how intent she was on making sure they heard the exclamation points in her tone. And, they heard them with all of the intent and instruction that they were meant to carry. I myself heard her message and was clear about the mission of end-of-life care for hospice patients. She cut away the fanfare and glory that we like to build into the great work of end-of-life care. She made it pragmatic and simple.

Elisabeth has been the deepest and richest nutrient—a formidable resource for nourishment—in the growth of hospice here in America. Whether the influence came from her books on death and dying, from her paradigm of the coping process, from the numerous interviews and tapes, or from her workshops and retreats, the message was clear, "LISTEN."

That "LISTEN" meant that there was no room for prearranged agendas when working with the dying. It meant not superimposing our own issues or concerns about death onto those we come to tend. It meant that whatever the patient brought up was what needed to be dealt with—even if it was difficult for us to deal with.

She clearly left some valuable tools in the end-of-life community. She showed us how to work with drawings. She offered keen advice on working with dying children. She taught us the value and meaning behind life. She opened us to crying and to laughing. She let us know that anger, denial, depression, bargaining, and acceptance were a part of many different emotional processes and that there was no order to the way in which we would feel them. She wrote and she wrote and she wrote some more.

She reminded us of the beauty of the butterfly. She shared how the cycle of the caterpillar's life is the cycle of birthing new ideas, emotions, or antechambers to the dwelling of our lives. She asked how could these small creatures adorn the walls of Bergen-Belsen, and Treblinka? What is the power in hope?

She deeply respected Viktor Frankl's works and always pushed his books on those who were around the dying and the dying process. She got me to read <u>Man's Search for Meaning</u> by her continued harping and her insistence on its ontological value. She actually shamed me into reading it. I had not read it after years of her prompting me to do so (on our monthly phone calls). When she asked me to come and visit her because she felt the end was near, I had still not read it. I gobbled up its powerful words on the plane to Arizona. I could not believe I had waited so long.

Above all of the things I learned from Elisabeth, it was the "LISTEN" that was most valuable. Not some passive form of checking out or zoning out while a patient opened themselves to telling of their stories—full of joy and pain. No, "attentive listening and feeling of what is being offered"; that is what she demanded, that is what she modeled.

This "LISTEN" was a serious and engaged process. The listening involved piecing the whole story together in a way that the teller may not be able do for themselves. It meant asking probing questions and waiting. It meant facing the raw images of each other's lives. It was fishing out the stories and tales of the journey—even when they were deep in the cool recesses of the heart's pools.

She has changed the way we die in America. She has given us great resources. She has taught us to "LISTEN" to the stories of our lives. And, she has reminded us not to be afraid; to wait for the unfolding of our wings as we emerge from life's many changes.

This very workbook was something she made me promise I would write. After sharing the format and the ideas with her, she told me to never stop trying to get it published; and to continue publishing articles on the work I had done with the dying and their families. She knew it would help professional caregivers to learn to listen in new ways.

Her greatest gift and greatest lesson was and is the same, "Listen". When we do, we will be surprised at how richly complex and dazzlingly robust life itself truly is. We will find dimensions that we had no idea were really there.

Afterword

To have completed any or all of this ***magnum opus*** is an immense accomplishment. There is a lot of material and ground that we cover in the ambling nature of our journey on this earth-place. You are to be commended. Getting it all out and onto paper is an awesome task.

You may have had to leave certain portions blank. I encourage you to go back, slowly, and add a little more over time. But, make sure you go back.

Sometimes small thoughts or feelings can achieve immense tasks—one emotion may sidetrack us from living our lives. A small diversion can take us on tangents that last a lifetime—or if not, a very long stretch of the road. I think we all have been on them before. We have all been derailed at some point.

The Talmud tells us that the smallest of hands, held before our eyes, can obscure the greatest of mountains from our view. My hope for you is that you will move whatever thoughts or feelings may be keeping you from completing any or all of this ***magnum opus***. Move them out of your life with the help of those who are providing you care and those who love you. Or, at least move them out of your life long enough to get some of this work done.

May you find the inner spark to pass on to your loved ones some of the stories that have made your life your own. May you return to this piece, again and again, until it is complete. May you gain nourishment from all that is held here; from all you have lived.

One of the things that hospice folks have learned from the work itself is, when we do life review—at any stage of life's journey—we gain a deepening strength and vilifying encouragement. It comes from seeing how complex our lives are, all of the places we have been, and all the difficulties we have overcome. We tend to forget these things in the short view of our lives. Life review helps plug us into the long view of our lives.

Gain courage from the long view. Share that courage with those you love.

www.ingramcontent.com/pod-product-compliance
Lightning Source LLC
Chambersburg PA
CBHW060506090426
42735CB00011B/2130